T0271777

WHAT IS SEX?

in the same series

What Is Pregnancy?
Kate E. Reynolds
Illustrated by Jonathon Powell
ISBN 978 1 78775 939 8
eISBN 978 1 78775 940 4

What Is Menopause?
Kate E. Reynolds
Illustrated by Jonathon Powell
ISBN 978 1 78775 941 1
eISBN 978 1 78775 942 8

by the same author in the *Sexuality and Safety with Tom and Ellie* series

What's Happening to Ellie?
Kate E. Reynolds
Illustrated by Jonathon Powell
ISBN 978 1 84905 526 0
eISBN 978 0 85700 937 1

Things Ellie Likes
Kate E. Reynolds
Illustrated by Jonathon Powell
ISBN 978 1 84905 525 3
eISBN 978 0 85700 936 4

What's Happening to Tom?
Kate E. Reynolds
Illustrated by Jonathon Powell
ISBN 978 1 84905 523 9
eISBN 978 0 85700 934 0

Things Tom Likes
Kate E. Reynolds
Illustrated by Jonathon Powell
ISBN 978 1 84905 522 2
eISBN 978 0 85700 933 3

What Is Sex?

A Guide for People with Autism, Special
Educational Needs and Disabilities

Kate E. Reynolds

Illustrated by Jonathon Powell

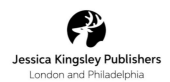

Jessica Kingsley Publishers
London and Philadelphia

First published in Great Britain in 2022 by Jessica Kingsley Publishers
An Hachette Company

1

A CIP catalogue record for this title is available from the British Library
and the Library of Congress

ISBN 978 1 78775 937 4
eISBN 978 1 78775 938 1

Printed and bound in China by Leo Paper Products

Jessica Kingsley Publishers' policy is to use papers that are natural, renewable
and recyclable products and made from wood grown in sustainable forests.
The logging and manufacturing processes are expected to conform to the
environmental regulations of the country of origin.

Jessica Kingsley Publishers
Carmelite House
50 Victoria Embankment
London EC4Y 0DZ

www.jkp.com

Thank you to my granddaughter, Mina Elizabeth Nancy, for making me a Nonna.

Kate

Many thanks to Geraldine Tartan for her love, support and encouragement.

Jonathon

DISCLAIMER

Illustrations and wording in this book are explicit and focus on aspects of sexuality and relationships. The author and illustrator are not responsible for any offense that may be caused.

The content of this book should not be regarded as a substitute for the advice of a medical or mental health professional practitioner or recommended therapy, treatment or professional consultation. The author and illustrator are not responsible or liable for any diagnosis made or actions taken based on the content of this book. Always consult your family doctor or licensed mental health professional if you are concerned about your health or that of a child or young person with autism, or other developmental and intellectual disabilities.

NOTES FOR PARENTS AND SUPPORT STAFF

This illustrated book uses explicit images and wording to explain sex. In health resources, sex is often alluded to, rather than being carefully explored with people with autism and special educational needs and disabilities (SEND). This may mean that they turn to online information of dubious quality, or pornography, which may warp their view of sex and relationships.

Many people with autism and SEND will have intimate relationships. To enhance the likelihood of them having positive relationships it is essential to discuss sexuality in the context of consent and sexual safety. For someone to consent they must have freedom and capacity to choose whether or not to have any form of sex. Having autism or SEND is not a reason to assume lack of capacity to make life decisions.

Knowledge of what constitutes sex is also an important part of preventing sexual abuse. This includes knowing proper names for sexual organs and sexual activities. Understanding sexual activity will help enable people with autism and SEND to refuse unwanted sexual advances from others and/or report it accurately.

People also need to know the possible physical consequences of having sex, notably pregnancy and sexually transmitted infections. Choices of contraceptive medication and barrier methods are explained briefly here but need full exploration by the person with medical professionals.

Each book in the *Healthy Loving, Healthy Living* series gives detailed information that can be read directly by individuals who have autism and SEND.

Sex is an important part of becoming an adult. It can be fun, exciting and make you feel really good. Sex is also a way of being close to your boyfriend or girlfriend. In this book we'll call them your partner.

Sex is sometimes called "sleeping with" your partner, but sex isn't sleeping. Sex is touching each other's bodies in different ways for pleasure. Sex is a private thing to do with your partner in a private place, like your own bedroom with the door shut.

Sex is kissing in an intimate way, perhaps putting your tongue inside your partner's mouth. This is different to the way you kiss your family and friends. Sex is touching each other's bodies through clothes. Sex is being naked with your partner and touching and enjoying each other's private body parts.

Some people wait to have sex until they are married or until they meet a special partner. Before you have any sex, you need to know what sex is and talk about it with your partner.

Wherever you live there is an age of consent. This means that you should not have any sex if you're under that age.

But you don't have to have sex if you're over the age of consent. It's up to you.

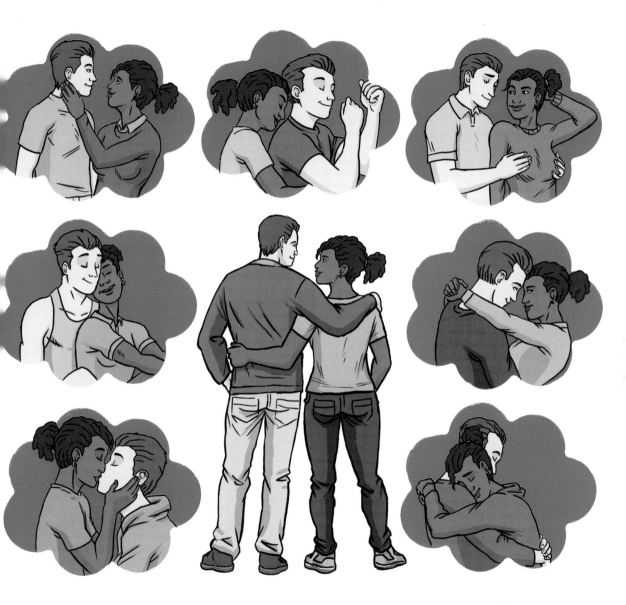

Men's breasts or chests are flat with nipples in the middle.

Men have a penis. Penises look different to each other. They can be thicker or thinner, shorter or longer, different colours and with different kinds of pubic hair, and can be straight or slightly bent.

Behind the penis is a bag of skin called the scrotum which has two ball shapes called testicles inside. They make sperm, which spurt out of the penis during sex.

Transgender men are physically women when they're born. These men sometimes wear a binder (like a small top but it's very tight) over their breasts until they have surgery to make their breasts flat, if they want to.

Transgender men may not have a penis or scrotum but these can also be made by surgery, if they want them. Medication can also help them look and feel more like men.

Men's buttocks look different to each other. The hole between the buttocks where poo comes out is called an anus.

If a man feels any lumps in his testicles, scrotum or anus he should see a doctor to make sure everything is okay.

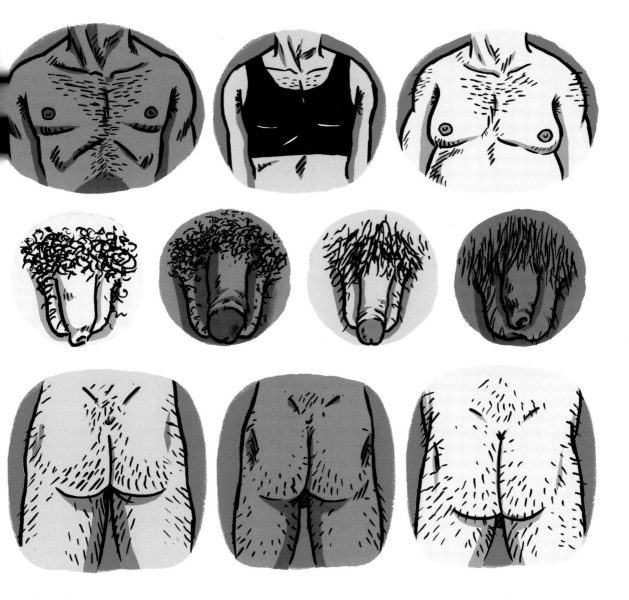

Women's breasts can be different shapes and sizes with a nipple in the middle. Some nipples stick out and others curve inwards.

Women have a vulva, which is at the front between the legs like a large pair of lips. Vulvas can be thinner or thicker, have a lot or not much hair.

Vulvas protect the clitoris (at the very front), the pee hole (in the middle), then the vagina, which is a hole that leads to the womb inside the body, where a baby would grow. A clitoris is very sensitive and it can feel very sexy and exciting when it's touched.

Transgender women are physically men when they're born. They may not have a vulva, clitoris, vagina and fleshy breasts until they have surgery, if they want to. They may feel and look more like women if they choose to take medication.

Women's buttocks look different to each other. They have an anus, where poo comes out, at the back between the buttocks and behind the vagina.

If the skin of a breast changes, nipples start to turn inwards from sticking out or a woman has lumps anywhere she should see a doctor to make sure everything is okay.

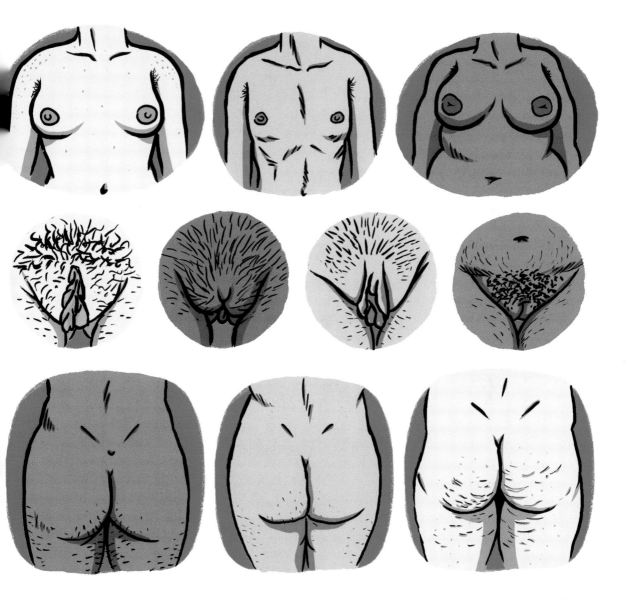

Consent to have sex means someone agrees (says yes) to have sex. You and your partner both have to agree to have sex together, not just one of you.

If you agree to have sex you can change your mind at any time.

If you are uncomfortable or not sure if you want to carry on, stop. Talk with your partner to tell them how you feel.

Saying "no" to sex doesn't mean the answer will always be no, but nothing has to happen until you're ready.

Agreeing to one type of sex doesn't mean you agree to have other types of sex. So if you kiss and hold your partner, this doesn't mean you agree to be naked with them.

Agreeing one time doesn't mean that you're saying "yes" to that kind of sex any other time, even with your same partner.

Sex isn't something that you owe your partner or they owe you. Sex won't stop your partner ending your relationship if they want to.

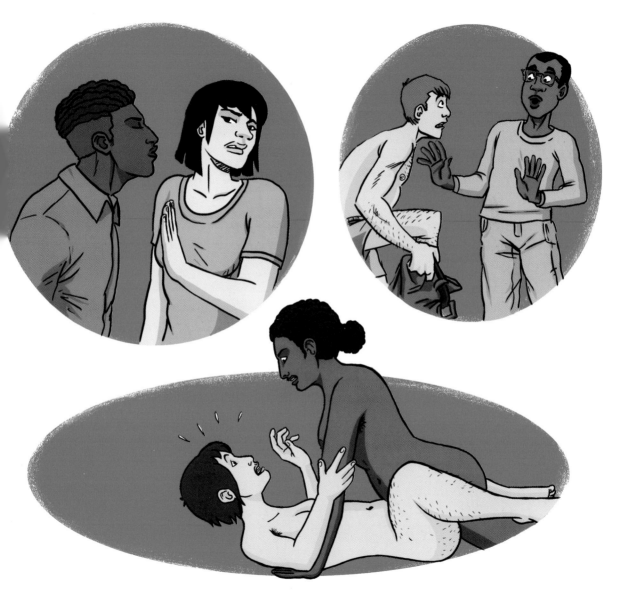

You can't agree to sex if you are:

- Drunk on alcohol.
- Drugged.
- Being forced to have sex by your partner.
- Too scared to say "no".
- Feeling under pressure to have sex, for example from friends.
- With a partner who is in authority over you, like a teacher or social worker.
- Under the age of consent.

Don't assume you have the consent of your partner. Like you, they can refuse at any time.

If your partner doesn't want to carry on having sex with you, they may become still or stiff. You need to stop straight away and check that they're okay.

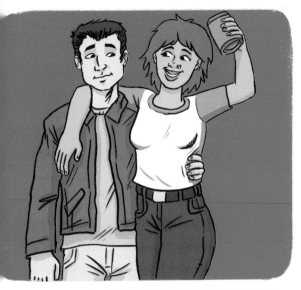
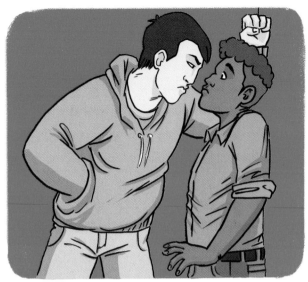
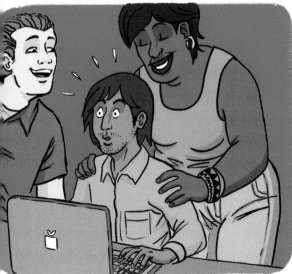
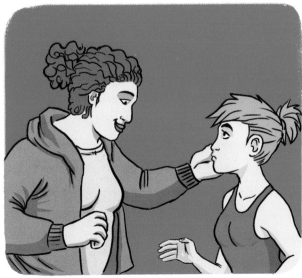

Foreplay is when partners do sexy things with each other, but don't actually have vaginal or anal sex. Vaginal sex is when sex involves a vagina; anal sex is when it involves the anus. You can feel closer and more relaxed with your partner by doing foreplay.

Foreplay might be:

- Kissing your partner's lips or body.
- Massage (rubbing the other person's body).
- Dry humping, which is making all the up and down movements of sex with clothes or underwear on. A partner may orgasm during dry humping.
- Fingering, when a partner uses their fingers to excite their partner's vagina or anus.
- Oral sex; although some people think this is sex rather than foreplay.
- Mutual masturbation.

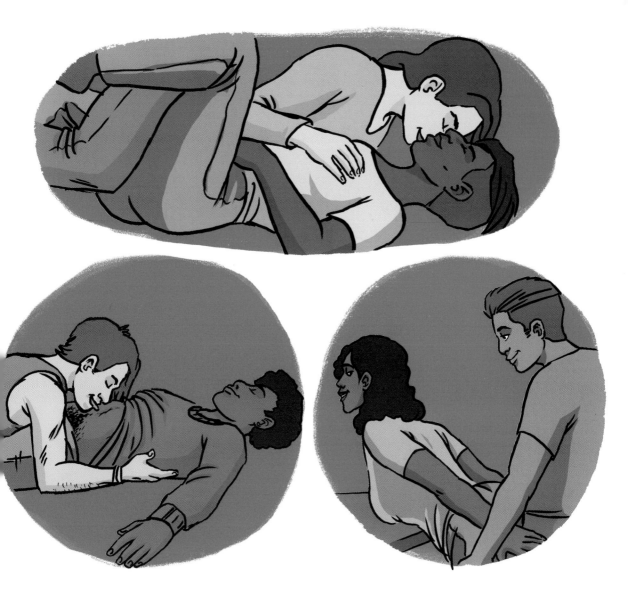

Mutual masturbation is when people rub and stroke their partner's private sexual body parts to get excited.

When a vulva, vagina and clitoris are excited by rubbing and stroking, the vagina can become wet.

A penis becomes hard and sticks out when it's excited.

Masturbation can be used before or during vaginal or anal sex to help your partner have an orgasm.

During an orgasm you and your partner become so excited that your heart and breathing get faster and you feel really happy.

Clear liquid can spurt out of a vagina when someone is having an orgasm and white liquid spurts out of the end of a penis.

This is also called ejaculating. It is different to urine or pee, which is yellow. After ejaculating it can take minutes or hours for someone's penis and testicles to return to their usual size, but it will happen.

You and your partner will often feel really relaxed and close after orgasms.

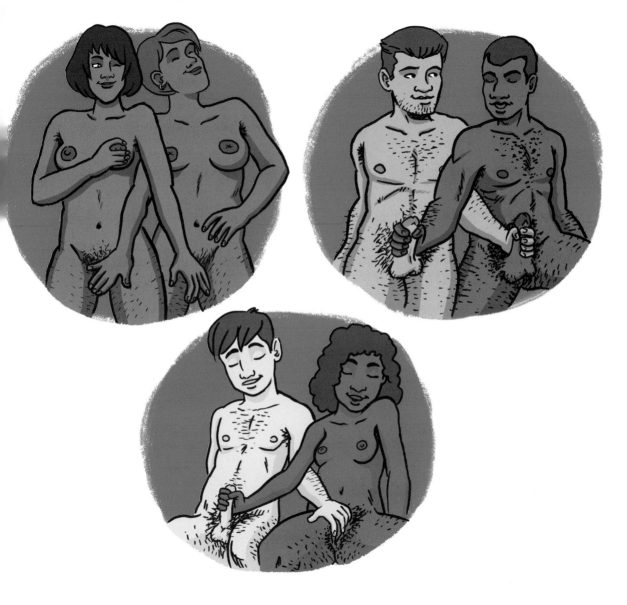

Oral sex is when someone uses their tongue, mouth and lips to lick or suck their partner's private sexual body parts.

A vagina, vulva and clitoris can be sucked and licked. This can make a partner orgasm and the vagina spurt liquid or become wet.

A penis and testicles can be sucked and licked. The penis can ejaculate or spurt semen when this happens.

An anus is very sensitive when sucked and licked.

You can get infections from doing oral sex, especially if you have any sores, ulcers or cuts in your mouth. Try not to brush your teeth just before oral sex because your gums might bleed. Use a mouthwash instead.

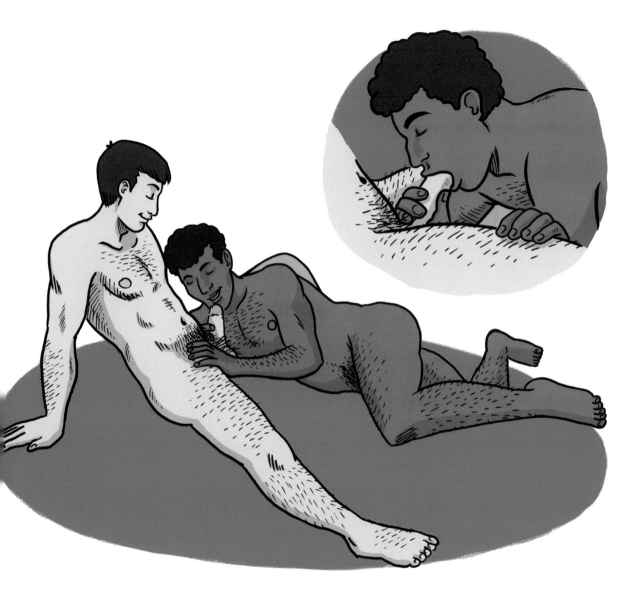

If you've done some foreplay with your partner, you might think about doing vaginal or anal sex. Talking with your partner will help you to both work out what you want or don't want to do.

Talking with your partner makes sex better, because you can tell each other what feels good and what you both really like.

You and your partner can also say if you feel unhappy, if something makes you feel uncomfortable or if you don't want to have sex.

If you're thinking of vaginal or anal sex it's a good idea to use lubricant. This should be water-based, which will be on the label.

Putting lubricant on your fingers and then into your partner's vagina or anus will make it easier for a penis or fingers to enter the hole.

Foreplay also helps your partner relax, which makes sex more comfortable and fun.

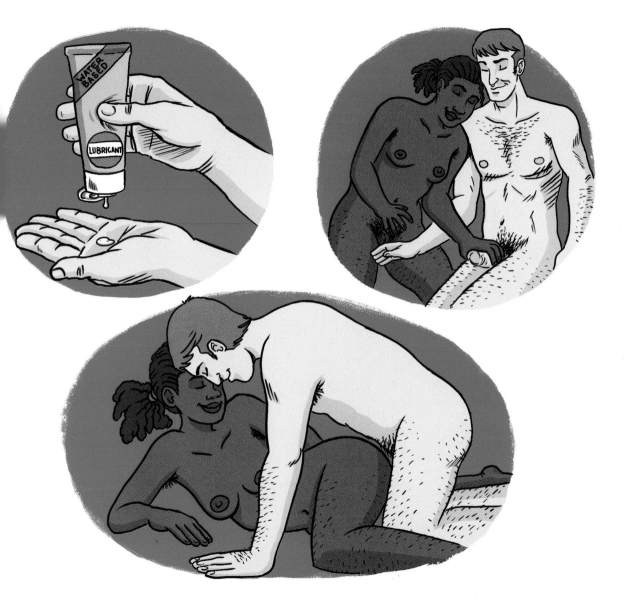

Vaginal sex is when a penis goes into a vagina during sex.

If a woman is a virgin it usually means she has not had vaginal sex before.

There is skin called a hymen, which partly covers the vagina. The first time a penis enters a vagina, the hymen may break and bleed a little and might hurt a bit. The hymen doesn't grow back.

Foreplay and lubricant help make the vagina wet, so sex is comfortable.

A penis has to be hard to go into a vagina.

When a man and a woman are having sex, the woman can be on top (like in the picture) or under their partner.

You can have vaginal sex when you're having a period, but you may want to put a towel underneath in case blood gets on your bed sheets.

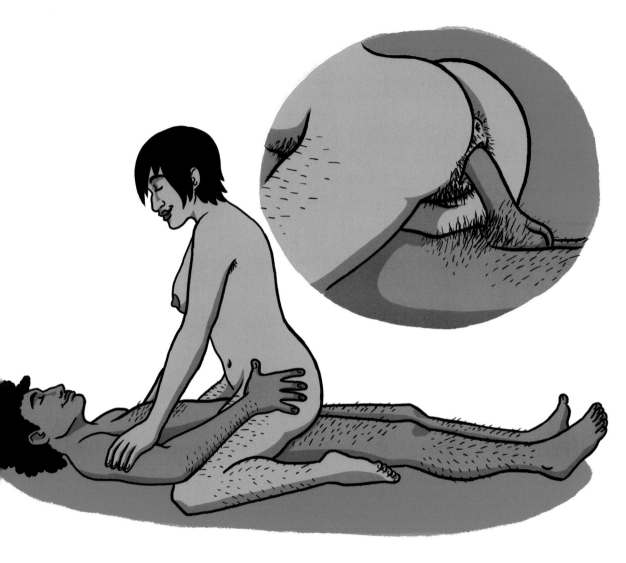

Anal sex is when the anus of a man or woman is sexually excited by having a penis put into it.

A penis has to be hard to go into an anus. If it's floppy, a penis will bend and won't go inside.

Anal sex can be painful and the anus may bleed a little unless lubricant is used to make it wet.

Foreplay, like fingering, also helps partners relax, which will make the anus easier for a penis to slide in.

Condoms make anal sex safer by preventing infections. Make sure you put on a new condom if you're having anal sex then going straight into doing vaginal sex. Otherwise you can pass infection from the anus into the vagina.

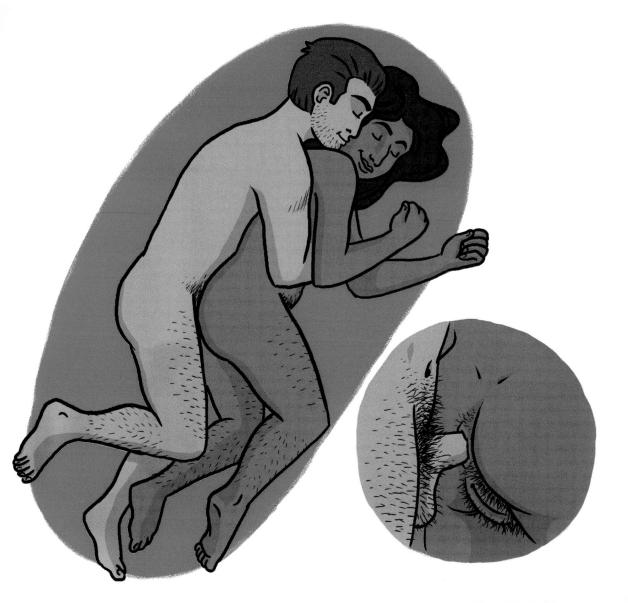

Vaginal sex can cause pregnancy. Semen from the penis contains sperm which look like tadpoles. If they join with a human egg inside someone who has a womb, a baby can grow there. This is called being pregnant.

If you don't want a baby, you have to use medicines called contraception. There are many types of contraception, like tablets or injections. You need to talk about these with your doctor, pharmacy or sexual health clinic to work out what is best for you.

Remember you can get pregnant:

- The first time you have vaginal sex.
- When you're having a period.
- If only part of a penis enters the vagina.
- Even if a penis is removed before it ejaculates or spurts semen.
- If there is semen on fingers when fingering a vagina.
- If there is semen near the vagina after anal sex.

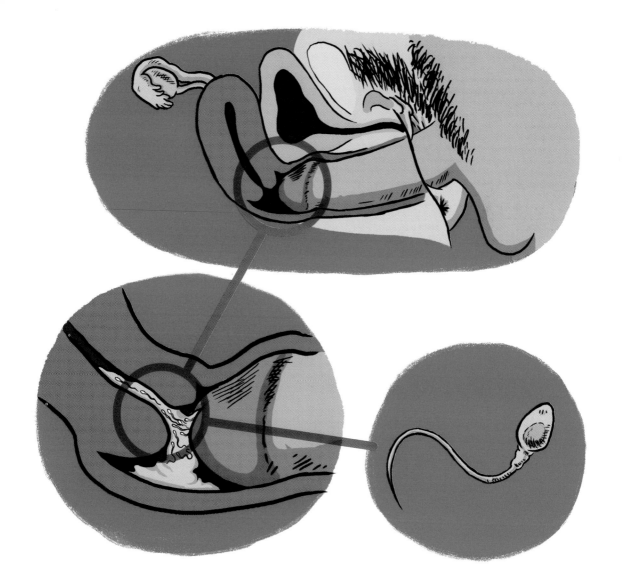

Sexually transmitted infections pass from one partner to another during sex. You can protect yourself by washing your hands before and after sex and using:

1. Condoms rolled fully onto a hard penis. Keep them on until the penis is pulled out after ejaculating or spurting semen. Condoms can be used for anal and vaginal sex. Flavoured condoms may be used for oral sex.

2. An internal condom that is put inside a vagina or anus. You can use lubricant to help slide it into place before sex happens. The rim of the internal condom sits on the outside of the vagina or anus.

3. Dams, which feel like condoms but are a flat square. They are often flavoured because you put them over a vagina or anus during oral sex, so your tongue licks through them.

You can practise putting condoms on or in before you're going to have sex, so you're not under pressure.

You can only use any condoms and dams once. Don't wash them out or use them again.

You can buy condoms and dams in pharmacies, from your doctor or in a sexual health clinic.

To stop infections and pregnancy, you should use contraceptive medicines and condoms or dams.

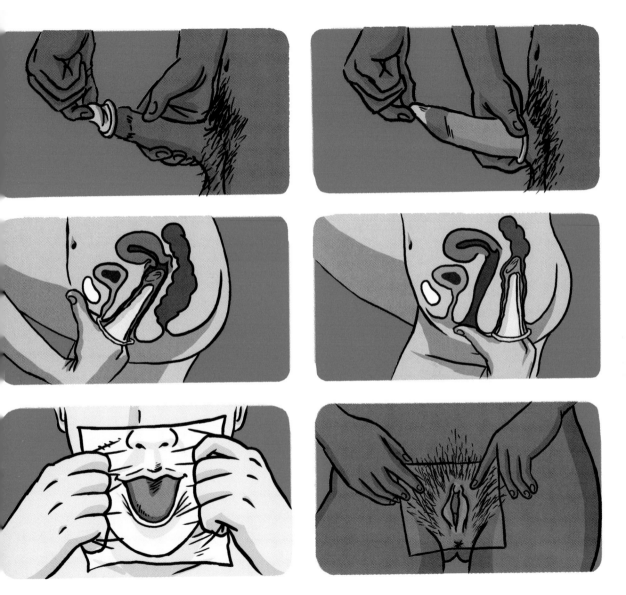

Having sex is a big step in your life and relationship. Sometimes it can help to talk about it with a person who isn't your partner.

Your doctor, pharmacy or sexual health clinic can give you advice about contraception or what to do if you think you're pregnant.

If you have discharge, itching, sores, blisters or lumps on your private body parts or pain when you're peeing, you might have an infection from sex. Sexual health clinics have experts who can find and treat these infections.

Medical professionals have to keep your confidentiality. That means they can't tell your parents or caregivers about your sex life unless you or someone else could be seriously hurt.

If you are forced to have sex, this is called rape or sexual assault and is against the law. You can report this to the police, a sexual health clinic, a doctor or someone you trust.

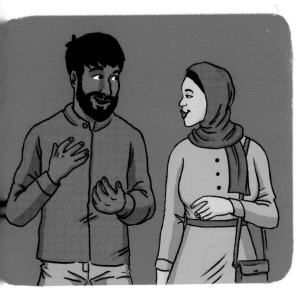
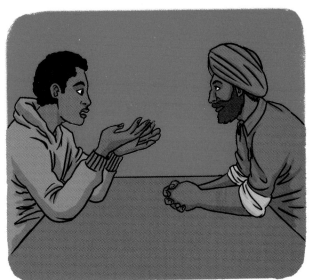
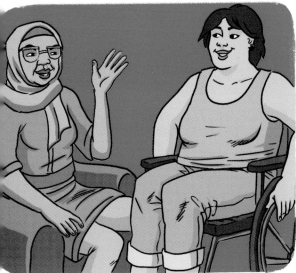
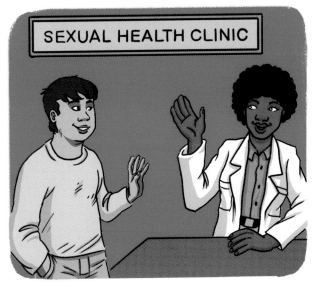

SEXUAL HEALTH CLINIC

WHAT SEXUAL HEALTH SERVICES ARE NEAR YOU?

It is a good idea to know what clinics and health centres are near you. You can visit them so you know exactly where they are, what they look like and how you get into the building. This might help you feel more confident if you need an appointment. Here's what the different health services can offer you.

Sexual health clinics usually tell you about different types of contraception and which might be right for you. They might check you for sexually transmitted infections (STIS) if you're worried about this.

Genitourinary medicine (GUM) clinics can also check you for different infections you can get by having sex.

Pharmacies can advise you and give you emergency contraception if your contraception hasn't worked or you had unprotected sex. You don't need an appointment to speak with the pharmacist. You can buy condoms and pregnancy tests at pharmacies without needing to speak to the pharmacist because they're on the shelves. They have instructions inside, but you may need a person you trust to help you use them.

Your family doctor can talk with you and refer you to other services.

Maternity services start after you have a positive pregnancy test.

Name of service and key person	Address and phone number of the service	What does the service do?	How to find the service
For example: Haven Women's Clinic. Keisha	**For example:** 58–59 High Street Soxley SX1 2GT 09876 543210	**For example:** Contraception advice	**For example:** Bus A12 to bus station. Walk across bridge. Clinic is grey building with white doors. Ring doorbell.

HOW TO MAKE AN APPOINTMENT

- Write down dates when you're free to have an appointment in the next few weeks. Write down your phone number because the service may text you with your appointment.
- When you ring, tell the person speaking to you what difference you have, such as autism. This helps them support you and give you more time, if you need it.
- If you prefer a woman or man doctor, you can say so. You don't have to say why you want an appointment, but it can help the person to work out how quickly to get your appointment.
- Write the appointment down immediately and repeat it back to the person on the phone so you get it right.

WHAT TO SAY AT AN APPOINTMENT

It's a good idea to write notes about what you want to ask because lots of people get nervous and forget what to ask. Think about:

- Asking who needs to know about your appointment, any tests and results. There may be people you don't want to know.
- Have you had some sort of sex? What happened? Did you consent (agree) to the sex you had? Did you use contraception?
- How to explain pain, itching or discharge from your penis or vagina and if it is getting worse, better or the same. How long have you had this?

WHO CAN YOU TRUST TO TALK TO?

Remember that people might have to tell someone else what you say, if they think you might hurt yourself or someone else.

Name and how you know them	Phone number	Address	How to meet them
Family **For example:** My sister Annie	**For example:** 01234 567890	**For example:** 63 Pleasant Mount, Boxton	**For example:** Train to Boxton Parkway. Annie meets me there.
Friends			
Support worker			
Social worker			
Teacher			
Helplines			

Kate E. Reynolds, MDS, PGDC, PGDHE, BSC (Hons) SA, RGN, is a mother to two children on the autism spectrum, one of whom has intellectual disabilities. She worked for the UK's National Health Service for 18 years, much of which was in HIV and sexual health. Kate has written 12 books, most published by Jessica Kingsley Publishers and almost all about aspects of relationships and sexuality. She works closely with parents, caregivers and health educators, as a public speaker, trainer, advisor and researcher.

Kate can be contacted through her websites at **www.kateereynolds.com** or **www.autismagonyaunt.com**

Jonathon Powell lives in Brisbane, Australia and has a Diploma in Fine Art and Bachelor of Animation from Griffith University, Queensland. He has illustrated for the *Sexuality and Safety with Tom and Ellie* six-book series by Kate E. Reynolds, *Can I tell you about Pathological Demand Avoidance syndrome?* by Ruth Fidler and Phil Christie and *Making Sense of Sex* by Sarah Attwood, all published by Jessica Kingsley Publishers. He provided artwork and animations for Family Planning Queensland (True). Jonathon also illustrated *What are... Relationships?* by Kate E. Reynolds.